EDITH CAVELL
A Legacy of Caring &]

Diana Souhami

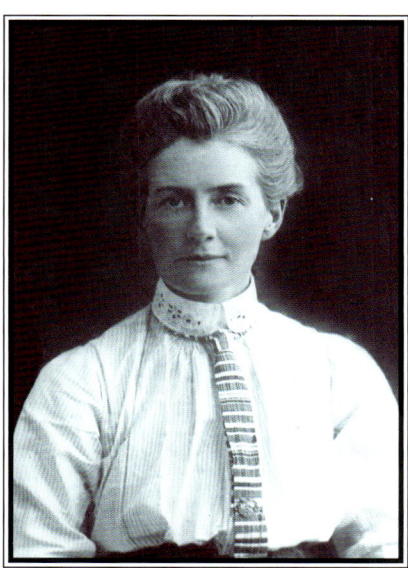

CONTENTS

Forewords	2
Prologue	4
Edith Cavell's Early Years	4
The Governess's Lot	6
Nurse Edith Cavell	7
The Brussels Matron	9
Edith Cavell's Character	10
Outbreak of War	11
Resistance Work	12
Watched & Sentenced	14
Remembered	19
Places to Visit	20

FOREWORDS

HRH The Princess Royal

BUCKINGHAM PALACE

I am delighted to be President of the Centenary Appeal for Cavell Nurses' Trust, the national charity which upholds Edith Cavell's living legacy of caring and learning and looks after all nurses, midwives and healthcare assistants in the UK if they experience hardship and distress.

This ethos is entirely in keeping with the aspirations of Edith Cavell, who had a vision for supporting nurses who had given a lifetime of care to others. The charity was established from public funds donated in the years following her death. This public support continues today in many ways, from the annual coffee mornings on International Nurses' Day to the more challenging prospect of climbing Mount Edith Cavell in Canada which is the focus of the Trust's Centenary Appeal.

In this book author Diana Souhami has vividly portrayed the life of Edith, from her Victorian childhood in a Norfolk vicarage to her courageous actions in saving hundreds of Allied soldiers before her execution in 1915. As a nurse in World War One Edith ensured that in the Red Cross hospital where she was Matron, her nurses cared for the wounded and sick of all nationalities. Edith's story still has the power to inspire us today and that is an honourable living legacy.

Anne

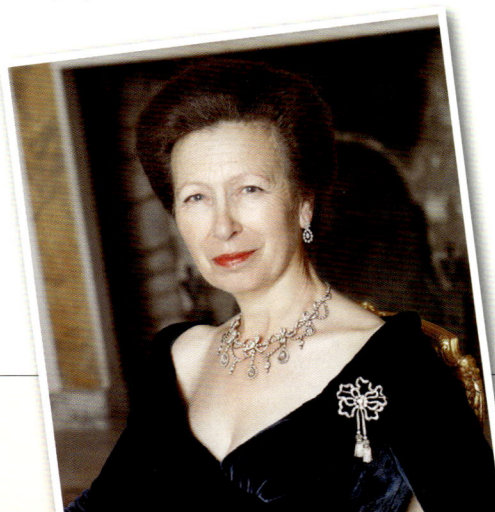

His Excellency The Belgian Ambassador
Mr Guy Trouveroy

Edith Cavell is known throughout Belgium for her courage, resolution, sense of duty and sacrifice. If you visit the Enclos des Fusilles in Brussels you will find her name on a memorial stone bearing the names of 35 heroes of the World War One resistance who gave their lives to protect others. Edith was executed at this place on 12th October 1915, together with four Belgian men.

Belgium will play a pivotal role in the international World War One centenary events planned over the next four years. As a country we have developed three central themes: collective remembrance; working together for a peaceful future; solidarity; and partnership. These are important themes which I feel Edith Cavell worked hard to fulfil during her lifetime; in setting up a nursing school in Brussels to improve professional standards; in the way she cared for soldiers in her wartime hospital, and in saving the lives of many Allied men.

We are proud to support Cavell Nurses' Trust throughout the centenary year and beyond, and commend the work undertaken by the Trust in keeping alight Edith Cavell's memory and her life's work.

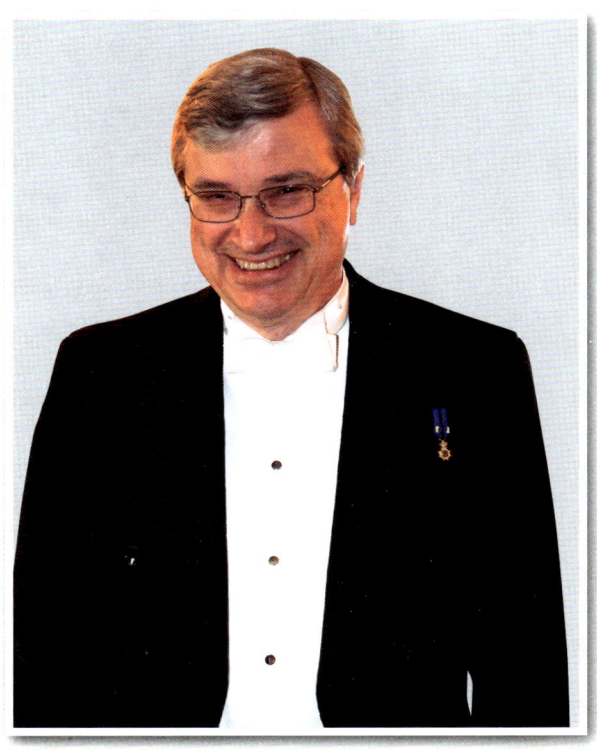

Prologue

On the evening of 11 October 1915 Edith Cavell was in cell 23 in St Gilles prison in Brussels. Armed German soldiers guarded the door. She had been in solitary confinement for ten weeks: no visits from a lawyer, priest or friends; no letters from home. She knew she was to be executed the next day.

At dawn she was taken to the city's shooting range, tied to a wooden post, blindfolded, shot by a German firing squad, and then buried without ceremony in a hastily dug grave. The officer who gave the command to the squad said they need have no qualms about shooting 'this woman'. He said she was not a mother and her crimes were heinous.

Edith Cavell's Early Years

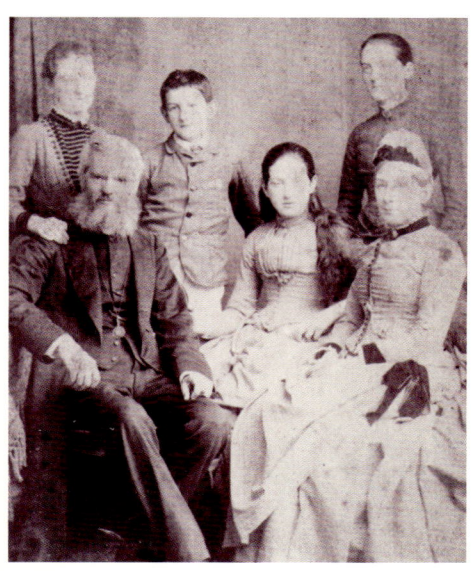

The Cavell family. Edith is at the back on the left. (Used with the kind permission of a Swardeston family whose forebears worked for the Cavell family)

Nothing in Edith Cavell's upbringing or background prepared her for the havoc and carnage of the First World War. She was born in 1865 in the Norfolk village of Swardeston, four miles from Norwich, into tranquil, time-honoured, English rural life. The village, sward and town, had a population of 350. Most of the land was owned by the lords of Swardeston Manor and Gowthorpe Hall. Villagers had very little. They handed down their trades and skills, father to son, married into each other's families and on marriage certificates often 'left their mark' in lieu of signature, for not many had been taught to write. They looked out for each other the way people in solid communities do. And although Edith Cavell in her life's work became extraordinary in her altruism and public service, her values were shaped by this ordinary, decent, peaceable living.

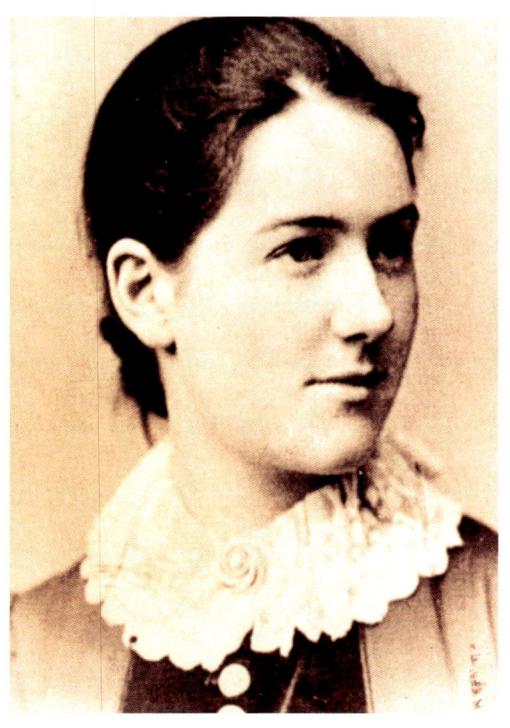

Edith Cavell as a teenager.

Her father was the vicar of Swardeston, a stern bewhiskered man, given to preaching dull sermons. He was the pivotal figure of village life and his influence on her was profound. From the cradle she was imbued with the duty to consider the welfare of others, share what she had, and to help those in need.

Reverend Cavell expected his children to be conformist and devout. Drummed into them was the necessity of salvation through prayer, obligation to the poor and contribution through service. Edith was the eldest child. A second Cavell daughter, born in 1867, was named Florence, after Florence Nightingale. A third daughter, Mary Lilian, followed in September 1870. All three became nurses. The birth of daughters was cause for thanksgiving but financial concern to the Reverend Cavell. Socially he was on a par with the squire; economically he was not much better off than the blacksmith. Sons were the breadwinners. Daughters were expected to be wives and mothers. The desired son and heir, John Frederick Cavell, was born in 1873. Named after his father and grandfather the expectation was for him to carry forward the family name, but he never married and in adult life took to the bottle. For thirty-two years he worked for the Norwich Union Insurance Company.

As a child, Edith Cavell found her father's orthodoxy repressive. In her teens she wrote to her cousin Edmund Cavell, 'I'd love you to visit, but not on a Sunday. It's too dreadful. Sunday School, church services, family devotions morning and evening. And father's sermons are so dull.'

She was educated at home until she was sixteen, then between 1882 and 1884 went to three different boarding schools in different parts of the country. Her father chose the schools through Church connections that offered financial concessions to the clergy. When Edith was nineteen she went as a pupil teacher to Laurel Court School, in the precincts of Peterborough Cathedral. Then, in 1887, Reverend Cavell found a post of governess for her with the family of Charles Mears Powell, vicar of Steeple Bumpstead, a small Essex village.

The Governess's Lot

To be a governess was one of the few work opportunities open to Victorian women who needed to earn money. It meant living in an unfamiliar house with an unknown family in return for a meagre wage and board and lodging. The governess, though childless herself, acted as a quasi-mother. She was a cut above the servants, but not of the family. It was a role derided in the literature of the time by writers like Charlotte Brontë. Socially it was a dead end. Edith Cavell's youth was not a time of coming-out balls and partying.

She spent a year with Reverend Powell and then, until she was twenty-five, worked as a day governess for wealthy families near her home. In 1890 she was recommended as a governess to Paul François, a Brussels lawyer with four children, who lived in Avenue Louise, a rich residential part of the city. It was an opportunity for Edith Cavell to live abroad, perfect her French, and work in a city that seemed as safe and civilised as Norwich.

She stayed for five years, got to know the city, and immersed herself in a new culture and language. There was much for her to enjoy: Paul François also owned a summer home in the Forêt de Longues near the Dutch border; she was respected and liked; she sketched and painted watercolours; but she felt unfulfilled. 'Being a governess is only temporary', she wrote to her cousin Edmund, 'but someday, somehow, I am going to do something useful. I don't know what it will be, I only know that it will be something for people. They are most of them so helpless, so hurt and unhappy.'

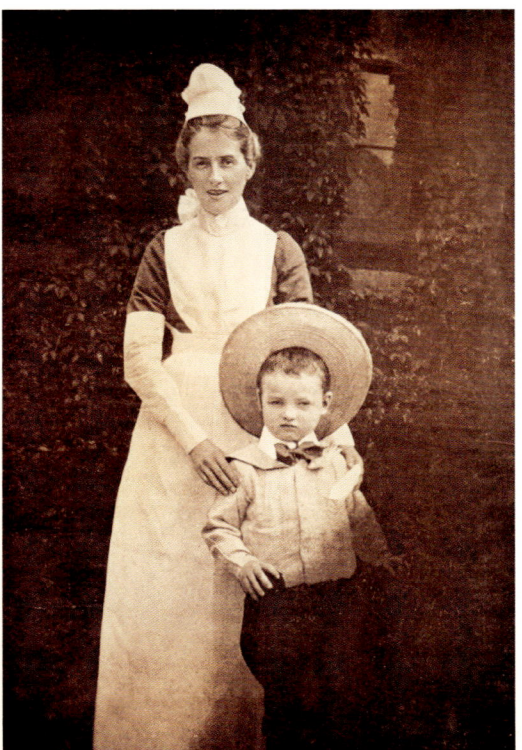

Edith Cavell with a young boy when she was assistant matron in Shoreditch.

Nurse Edith Cavell

Nursing was the something useful, something for people thing she did. She returned home and started, at the age of thirty, as an assistant at the Fever Hospital in Tooting. Infectious diseases decimated and terrified Victorian communities: typhus, typhoid fever, cholera, smallpox, tuberculosis, influenza and diphtheria. There was no infrastructure for clean water or sanitation, no organised immunisation, no antibacterial drugs, no antibiotics. Patient survival depended on nursing efficiency and the drive to restrict contagion: isolation hospitals, clean linen, much washing with carbolic, bedpans treated with disinfectants, rooms fumigated with sulphur.

After seven months she signed on as a probationer for formal nursing training at the flagship London Hospital. The matron there, Eva Luckes, a friend of Florence Nightingale, became her role model. Throughout her working life, Edith Cavell corresponded with her and sought her advice. All three women were reforming hospital matrons concerned with the universal application of best nursing practice. All had idealistic and demanding views about professionalism in nursing and, though themselves religious, wanted nursing to be secular, with proper pay and working conditions.

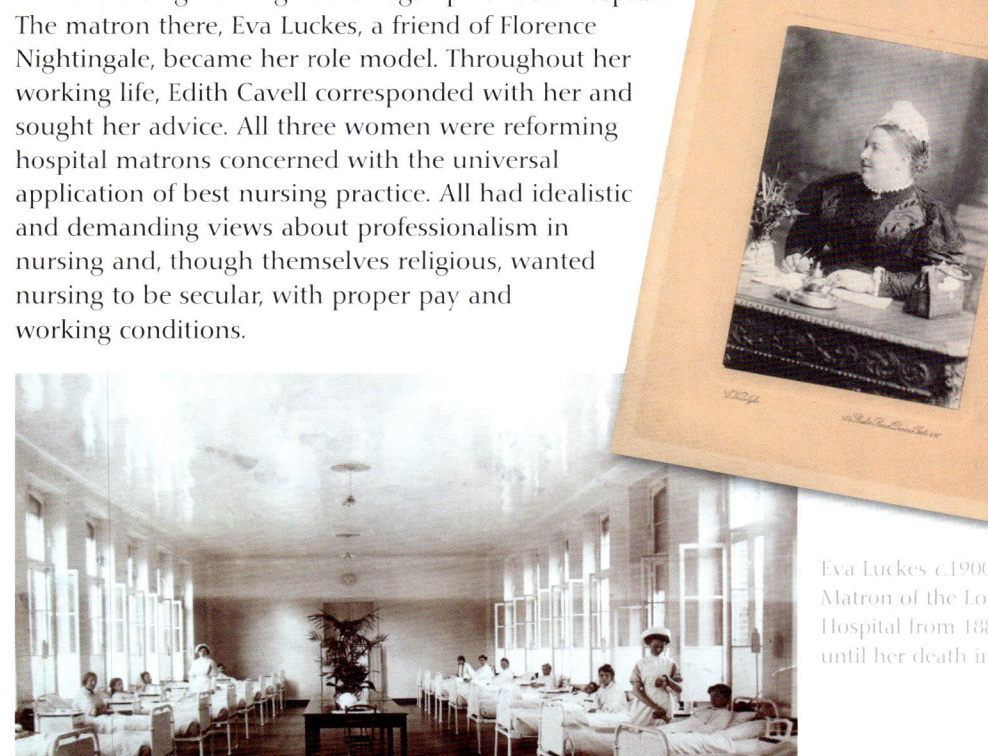

Eva Luckes c.1900, Matron of the London Hospital from 1880 until her death in 1919.

A typical Nightingale-style hospital ward in Edith's time.

While still a probationer, Edith Cavell nursed through a typhoid epidemic in Maidstone in Kent. In a graphic account of this epidemic the town's chief medical officer in 1897 wrote eloquently about the drains attached to the town's 4,000 water closets: 'each of which is nothing better than an elongated cesspool charged with foul festering filth that is perpetually producing air polluting and disease provoking vapours …'

One impetus for Victorian social reform came from the realisation that even if a typhoid epidemic began because the poor lived in squalor without proper sanitation, the rich man in his palace got a sore throat too. People became aware that if infection was to be contained there needed to be cohesive interaction between epidemiologists, bacteriologists, water companies, plumbers, governments and inspectors.

Patient survival depended on quality nursing. Edith Cavell worked to the highest standard of diligence and care. Were she to return today she would marvel at our infrastructures and technology; our plumbing, anaesthetics, antibiotics, vaccines and magnetic resonance imaging. She would see such things as marvels, putting heaven on earth in our reach.

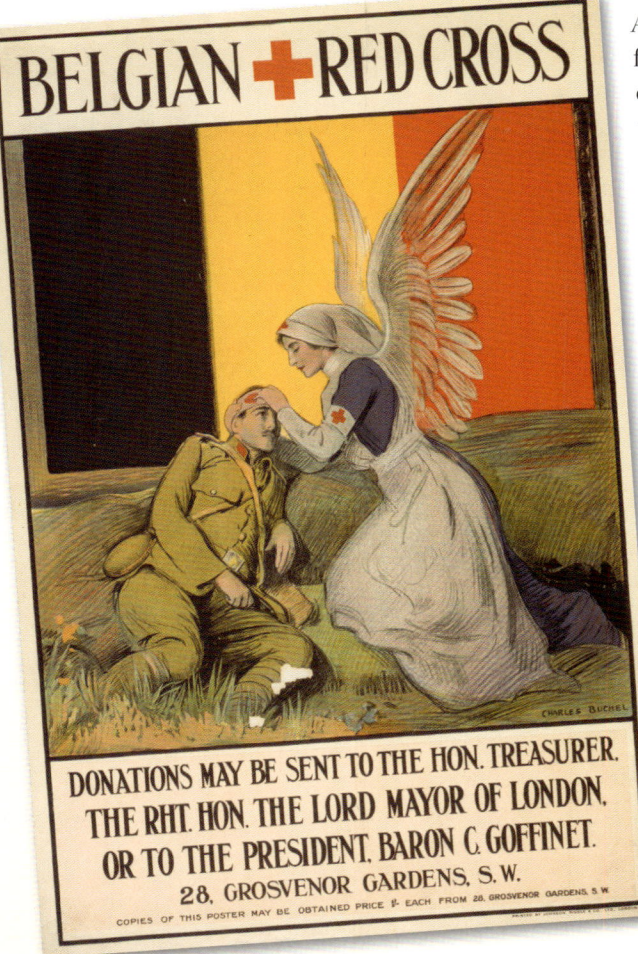

After she qualified she worked for a decade in different branches of nursing: as a staff nurse on various wards at the London Hospital; as a private nurse in people's houses; for three years as a night superintendent at the St Pancras Infirmary in London (the infirmaries evolved from the workhouses and were catch-all places for the impoverished sick – one in five patients died); then as an assistant matron.

Left: Belgian Red Cross poster.

Opposite: Edith Cavell and her student nurses at the École d'Infirmières Diplômées in Brussels.

The Brussels Matron

Edith gained wide nursing experience, but she wanted to be a matron and to make structural change. Her major career opportunity came in 1907 when she was invited by Belgium's leading surgeon, Antoine Depage, to go to Brussels as head matron of his clinic and start up a secular training school for nurses on the lines of Eva Luckes's at the Royal London Hospital. The intention was to revolutionise hospital provision in Belgium. Before Edith Cavell went out there, nursing in Belgium was by untrained nuns, of no particular competency – much like nursing in Britain before Florence Nightingale's reforms. Her work over the next eight years, until her arrest in 1915, was truly impressive and her diligence in setting up the school unremitting. She oversaw the care of patients, nurses and probationers, instructed domestic staff, planned and implemented projects with Depage, interviewed prospective nurses, gave lectures to the nurses, did all the administrative work and accounting, and assisted the surgeons during operations. Her school became the benchmark for nursing standards in Belgium. By 1912 Edith Cavell had trained nurses for three hospitals, three private nursing homes, twenty-four schools, and thirteen kindergartens in Brussels.

It was a measure of the esteem in which she was held that under her watch as matron a new, state-of-the-art nurses' training school and hospital had been funded, approved and was being built. However, in 1914 the First World War begun.

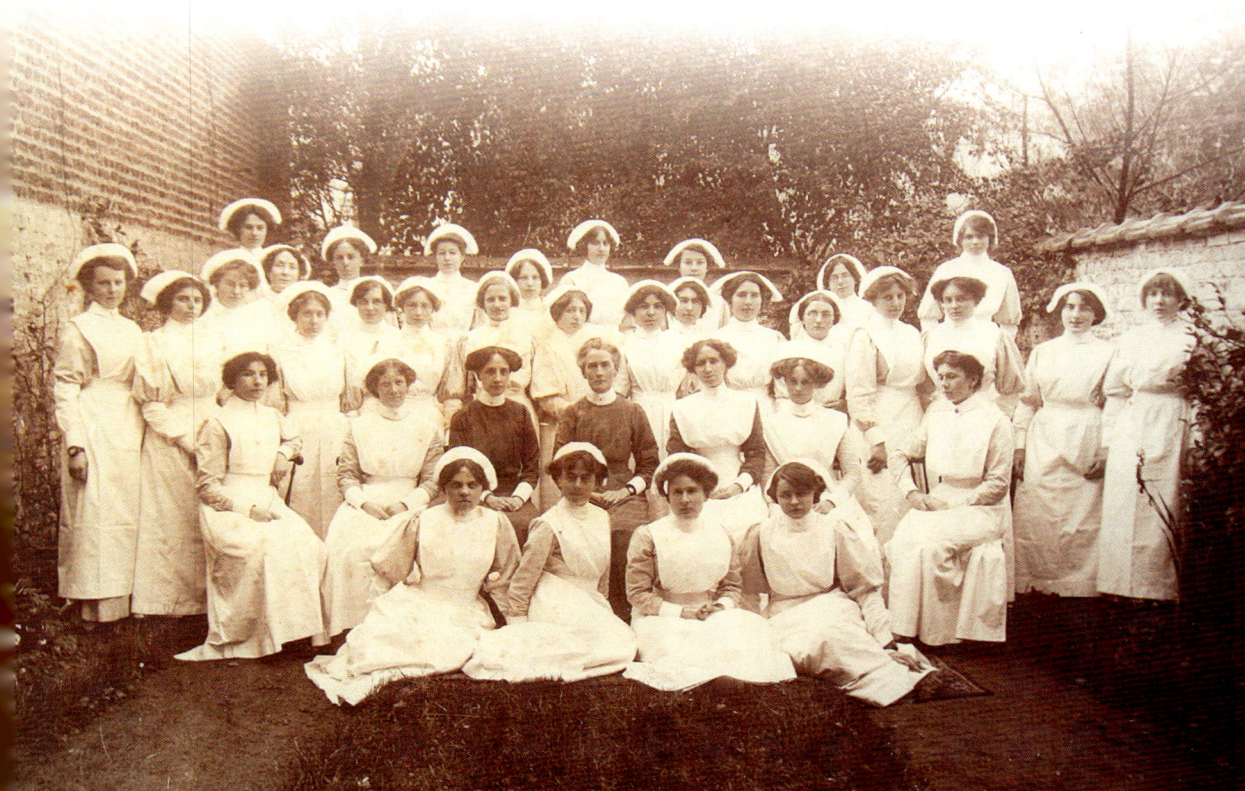

Edith Cavell's Character

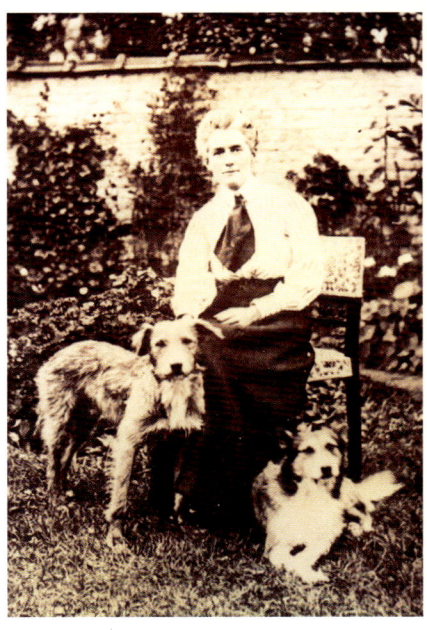

Altruism was Edith Cavell's defining quality – as a nurse, as a woman and, by chance, as a resistance worker. She thought invariably about what she could do to make life better for those around her rather than about profit or prestige for herself. She was truly a public servant.

She was slight in build, five foot three inches tall, with grey eyes and brown hair. She was quietly spoken and reserved in manner. Even in civilian clothes she looked as if she was in uniform. Navy blue was her colour. She viewed indiscipline as unprofessional, but her sternness was in order to achieve excellence at the training school: she insisted that her nurses wear their caps centred with their hair tucked back – they liked to wear them at an angle. At mealtimes she sat with a watch beside her plate at the head of the table in the nurses' dining room. Latecomers forfeited time off.

Edith Cavell with her dogs Don and Jack.

Early photographs show her to be not round, but not thin. In a photograph taken the year she died, she looked gaunt. An inventory of her possessions, taken after her death, was striking in its frugality: a suitcase of clothes, some books, a tea service, a paint box, a sketch pad, a camera … But though her aspect was restrained, the motivation of her life was sublimely romantic. As a Christian she believed heaven on earth could be achieved if all people did their best. As a nurse she believed that in time, with the best medical practice, disease would be eliminated.

Nor was she unremittingly stern. Even before the outbreak of war aspects of her life were fearlessly unconventional. At the school she created an oddball family. It began with the arrival of Jack the mongrel dog. He arrived at the back door, was given a meal, and from then on would not let Edith Cavell out of his sight. Jack is now stuffed and resides in the Imperial War Museum in London.

Pauline Randall, the thirteen-year-old daughter of a travelling circus owner, had a permanent place at the school; her mother was dead and her father abusive. Edith Cavell took her in and became her godmother. She also gave parental care to Grace Jemmett, a permanent patient with mental health problems and a morphine addiction. Sister Elisabeth Wilkins, the school deputy, became Edith Cavell's devoted friend.

Outbreak of War

Saturday 1 August 1914 was a defining day for Edith Cavell and for the world. She was in Norfolk for her summer holiday. She always made sure she went home for her mother's birthday in July. Her mother was by then widowed and living in a small terraced house in Norwich. The news in the papers was of a heatwave and trouble in the Balkans. That afternoon Edith Cavell visited her friends, the Blewitt sisters, who lived in the old rectory next to the vicarage in Swardeston. They had tea in the garden in the shade of the cedar tree on the lawn by the lake. The scene was the quintessence of peacetime: late summer, the calm of an English garden. There was no sense of it being a last summer or that politics might bludgeon its way into this time-honoured, civilised life.

In view for Edith Cavell was all that had informed her childhood: the church, the vicarage, the lake where she swam in the summer and skated in the winter. And all around were the lanes and fields of the England she knew, the landscape to which she returned each year because it was home, the place to where she intended to retire when old.

And then a maid brought out a telegram from Sister White at the school in Brussels. It was about the expectation of war and concern as to how their matron would manage to return. A week later nineteen million men were under arms in Europe.

Edith Cavell hurried back to Belgium thinking she would be more than ever needed as a nurse. On 20 August 1914 she watched as fifty thousand German troops marched into Brussels. The German plan was to march through Belgium and take Paris. These young soldiers were conscripts from towns and villages. Some, too exhausted to eat, slept on the pavement. When they took off their boots their feet were bleeding. Edith Cavell wrote that she felt 'caught between pity for these fellows, far from their own country, and hatred of a cruel vindictive foe, bringing ruin and desolation on hundreds of happy homes in a prosperous and peaceful land'.

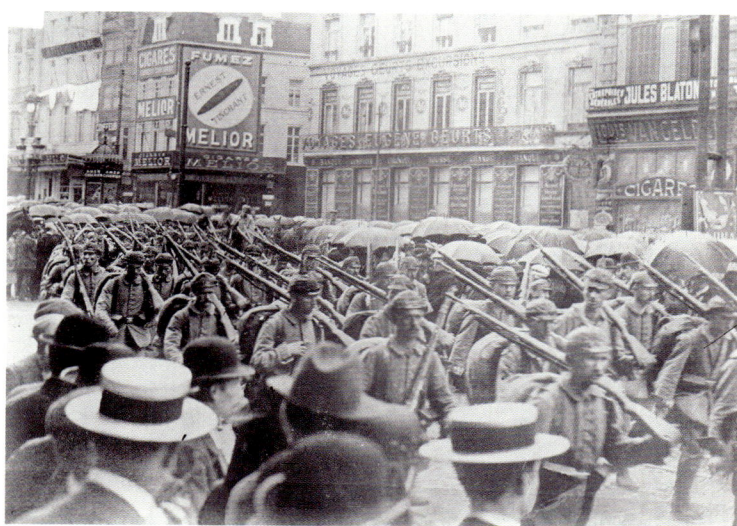

German infantry march into Brussels watched by civilians. Place Charles Rogier, 20 August 1914.

Resistance Work

Edith did not set out to be a resistance worker. She was a nurse. Her intention was to care for those wounded in the war. She told her nurses they must not take sides in the conflict. Their work was for humanity. Any wounded man, she said, must be medically treated; each was equal at the point of need. Each man was a son, husband, or father. But the occupying German military imposed restrictions on her opportunity to nurse. They set up hospitals for their own wounded and dispatched captured Allied soldiers to hospitals and prisoner-of-war camps in Germany.

Much of the First World War was fought in fields and trenches in Belgium and France. After battles such as that at Mons, where the German army won, wounded Allied soldiers became separated from their regiments. They hid in woodland or sought help from villagers. If captured they were shot or sent to prisoner-of-war camps in Germany.

The Belgians called these men 'enfants perdus', lost children. Edith Cavell did not go out looking for them, but when two wounded English soldiers were secretly brought to her clinic, she nursed and sheltered them. She then provided them with false papers,

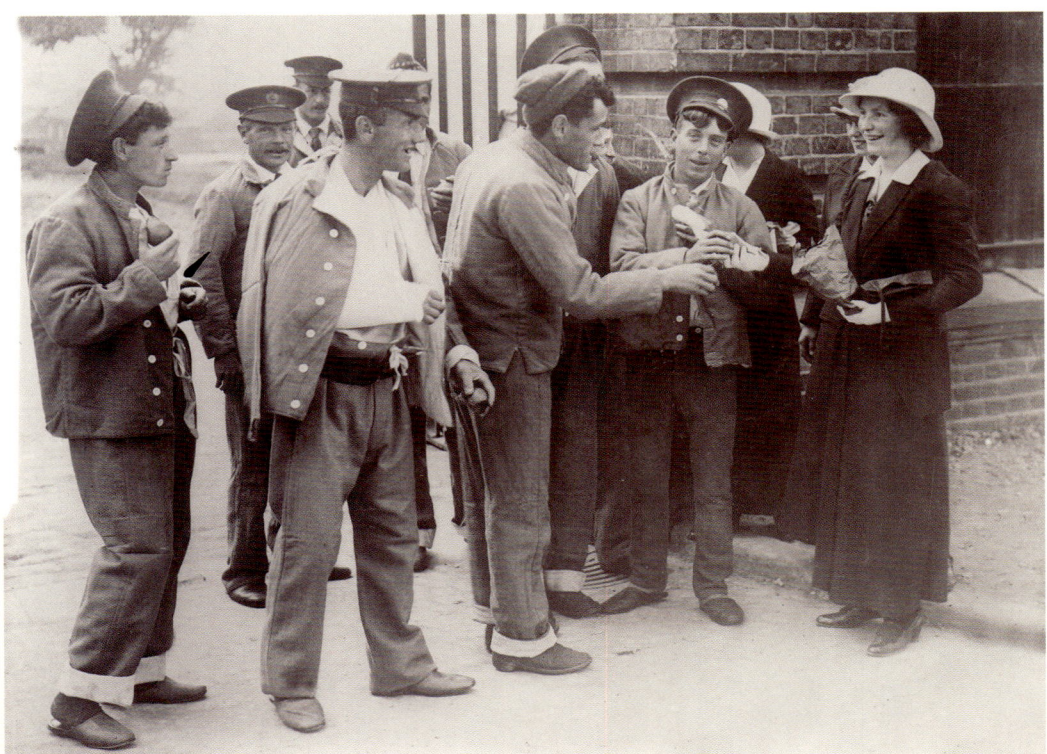

Wounded heroes of the Battle of Mons, 1914.

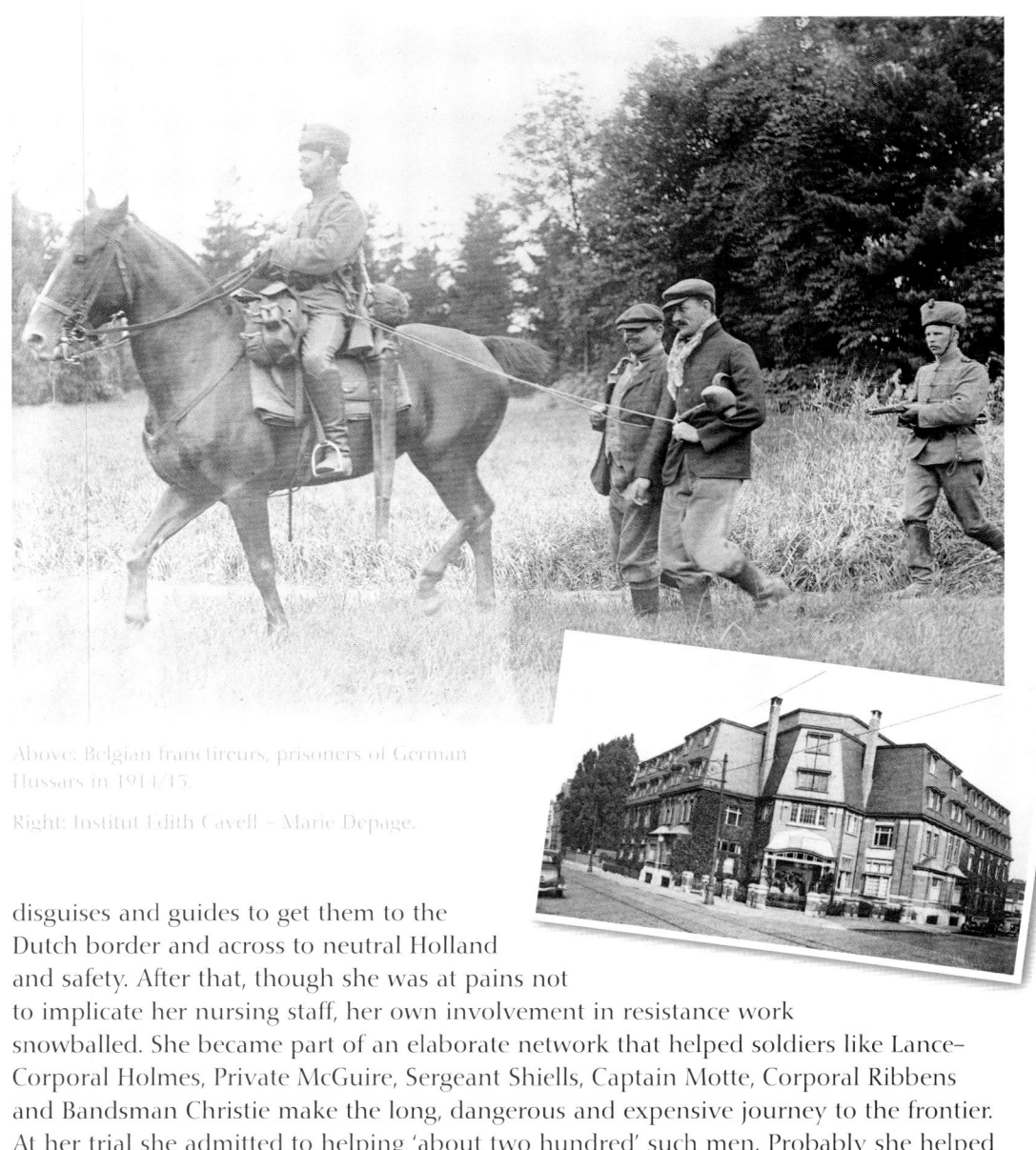

Above: Belgian franctireurs, prisoners of German Hussars in 1914/15.

Right: Institut Edith Cavell – Marie Depage.

disguises and guides to get them to the Dutch border and across to neutral Holland and safety. After that, though she was at pains not to implicate her nursing staff, her own involvement in resistance work snowballed. She became part of an elaborate network that helped soldiers like Lance-Corporal Holmes, Private McGuire, Sergeant Shiells, Captain Motte, Corporal Ribbens and Bandsman Christie make the long, dangerous and expensive journey to the frontier. At her trial she admitted to helping 'about two hundred' such men. Probably she helped a thousand. Her network arranged safe houses, passwords, bribes, guides, and ever-changing paraphernalia of codes.

Many women as well as men in Belgium, outraged by Germany's invasion of their country, laid their lives on the line to resist occupation. Edith Cavell's network included a French teacher, Louise Thuliez, her friend Henriette Moriamé, who after the war became a nun, and an aristocrat Jeanne de Belleville. They would walk twenty-four miles in a night, searching ditches and woodland to find these lost wounded men and get them to safety. The network was headed by the Prince de Croÿ who had high-level diplomatic connections in Britain and was a cousin of the Belgian King.

Watched & Sentenced

Edith Cavell and her network were watched. Thousands of casual spies, informers and agents provocateurs were in the pay of the secret police – about 6,000 in Brussels by the spring of 1915. They rode on trams, intercepted post, gave bribes and turned civilians over to the military courts, prisons and firing squads. Edith Cavell, fearful of turning genuine freedom-seekers from her door, erred on the side of trust. Knowing she and her network were under suspicion, she burned papers and records. She was finally trapped by Georges Gaston Quien, who called at the clinic and told her he was an officer wounded at Charleroi and needed to get to Holland.

She was interrogated by Lieutenant Bergan and Sergeant Pinkhoff who headed espionage in Brussels. Bergan put questions to her in German, which she did not speak; Pinkhoff translated these questions into French and Edith Cavell's answers into German. The deposition she signed was in German. She had no way of knowing whether it was what she had said.

Thirty-five accused were tried before a military tribunal. Edith Cavell had no proper defence lawyer. It was a kangaroo court. She was indicted for working 'to transmit soldiers into the ranks of the allies'. She expected imprisonment, but because she was English she inspired special hatred amongst the German military. She and a Belgian architect called Philippe Baucq were sentenced to death. Others in the network were sent to prisoner-of-war camps. The Prince de Croÿ escaped to England.

The cell to which Edith Cavell was confined at St Gilles prison was two and a half metres wide and painted white. There was a bed that folded into a table, a gas lamp, a chair and a bucket for a toilet. Food was passed through a wicket door.

She had writing paper, a pen and ink, her prayer book and a copy of Thomas A. Kempis's *Imitation of Christ*. She scored lines against texts that gave her courage to face her ordeal: the exhortation not to fear the judgement of men if her conscience was clear; to accept without bitterness what she could not change; to stay true to what she believed about goodness and love and not to give way to rancour or despair. 'Vanity it is to wish to live long and to be careless to live well' was one of his texts she highlighted.

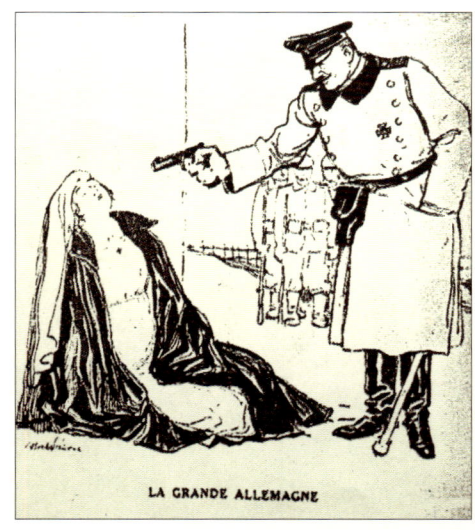

Cartoon of Edith's execution.

Diplomatic efforts in Brussels and London to save her were tardy and ineffectual. On the afternoon of 11 October 1915 the German pastor of the prison told her she was to be executed the next morning. He said he would try to arrange for her priest, the Reverend Stirling Gahan, from the Anglican church where she worshipped in Brussels, to call and give her Communion. By 8 p.m. he had not arrived and she had given up hope of his coming.

To give courage to her nurses at the school, Edith Cavell wrote them a letter of farewell in which she summed up the achievements of the eight years of her directorship of the school: how everything had been new at first, even the vocabulary; how the premises had not been fit for purpose; and at the start there had only been four probationers, but then, as dozens of nurses qualified, they had built up one service after another throughout Belgium, and now a new, state-of-the-art hospital and nurses' training school was nearly completed. 'When better days come our work will again grow and resume all its power for doing good,' she wrote. 'In your new beautiful Institute you will have more patients and all that is necessary for their comfort and your own.' She was, she told her nurses, more concerned about them and the new school than her own fate.

Ten hours before she was to be killed the Reverend Gahan arrived at the prison. A German guard let him in when he proved he had dispensation to see Edith Cavell. The guard said of her that she was a fine woman. 'Like this,' he said, and stiffened his back.

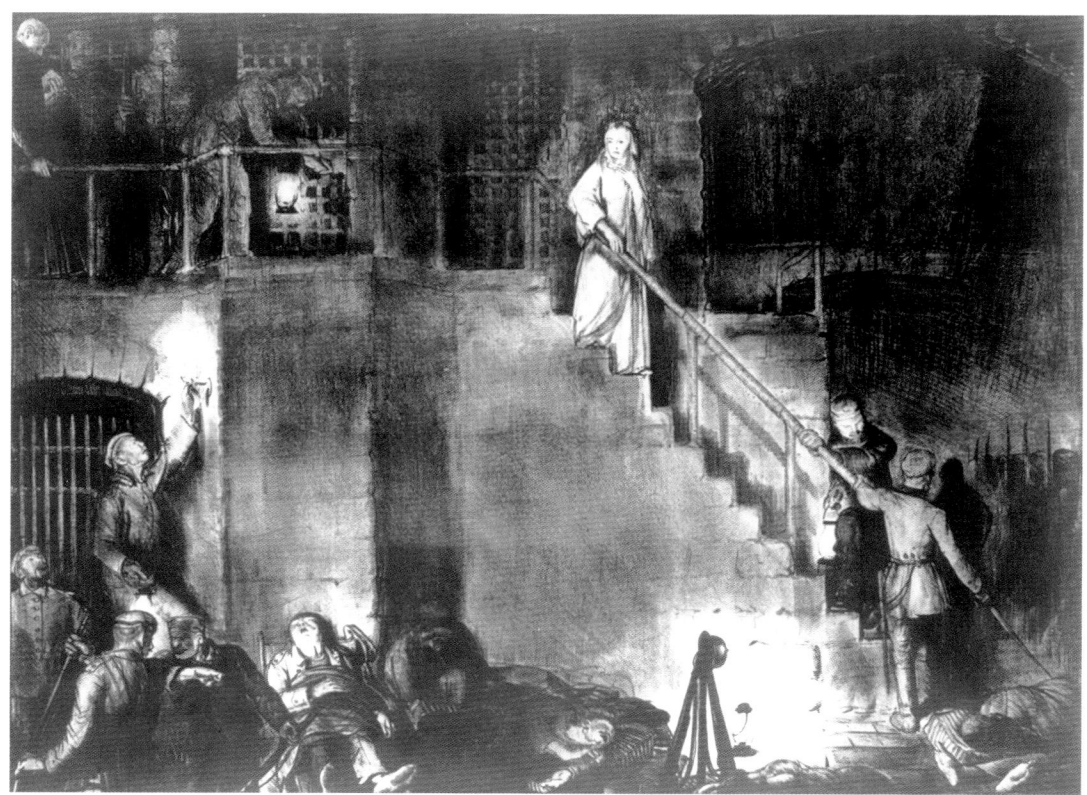

Murder of Edith Cavell by George Bellows, 1882–1925, artist.

Edith Cavell was in her dressing gown. Gahan had with him a silver Communion set. He had been apprehensive about her state of mind. On seeing her he was reassured. She told him it was good of him to come and gestured to him to sit on the one wooden chair.

She did not complain about her trial. She did not know that others who had stood trial with her and whose involvement in resistance work had been greater would be shown clemency. She said she willingly gave her life for her country and she described her imprisonment as 'a time of rest, a great mercy'. She told Gahan: 'Everyone here has been very kind. I have no fear or shrinking. I have seen death so often that it is not strange or fearful to me.'

The ritual of Communion linked her to her childhood in Swardeston, to the church visible from the rooms of the vicarage where she grew up, to her stern father and devoted mother, to the career decisions she had made, to her country which she looked to as a liberator from the injustice of a brutal occupation.

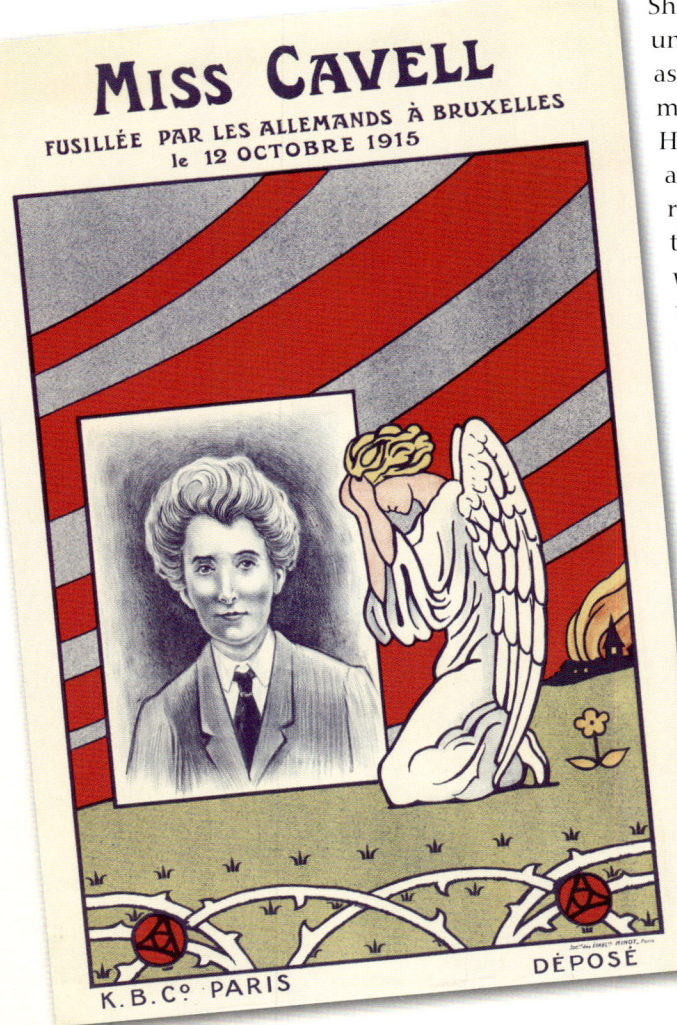

Miss Cavell shot by the Germans in Brussels, 12 October 1915.

She spoke to Gahan of her uncertainty about heaven and asked him to send farewell messages to friends and relations. He said, 'We shall remember you as a heroine and a martyr.' She replied, 'Don't think of me like that. Think of me as a nurse who tried to do her duty.' And then she spoke the words, part of which are engraved on the monument to her in Trafalgar Square: 'Standing as I do in view of God and Eternity I realise that patriotism is not enough. I must have no hatred or bitterness towards anyone.'

Gahan stayed with her for an hour and then said, 'Perhaps I had better go. You will want to rest.' She replied with her dry humour, 'Yes, I have to be up at 5 a.m.' She asked him to give to the prison's assistant governor letters

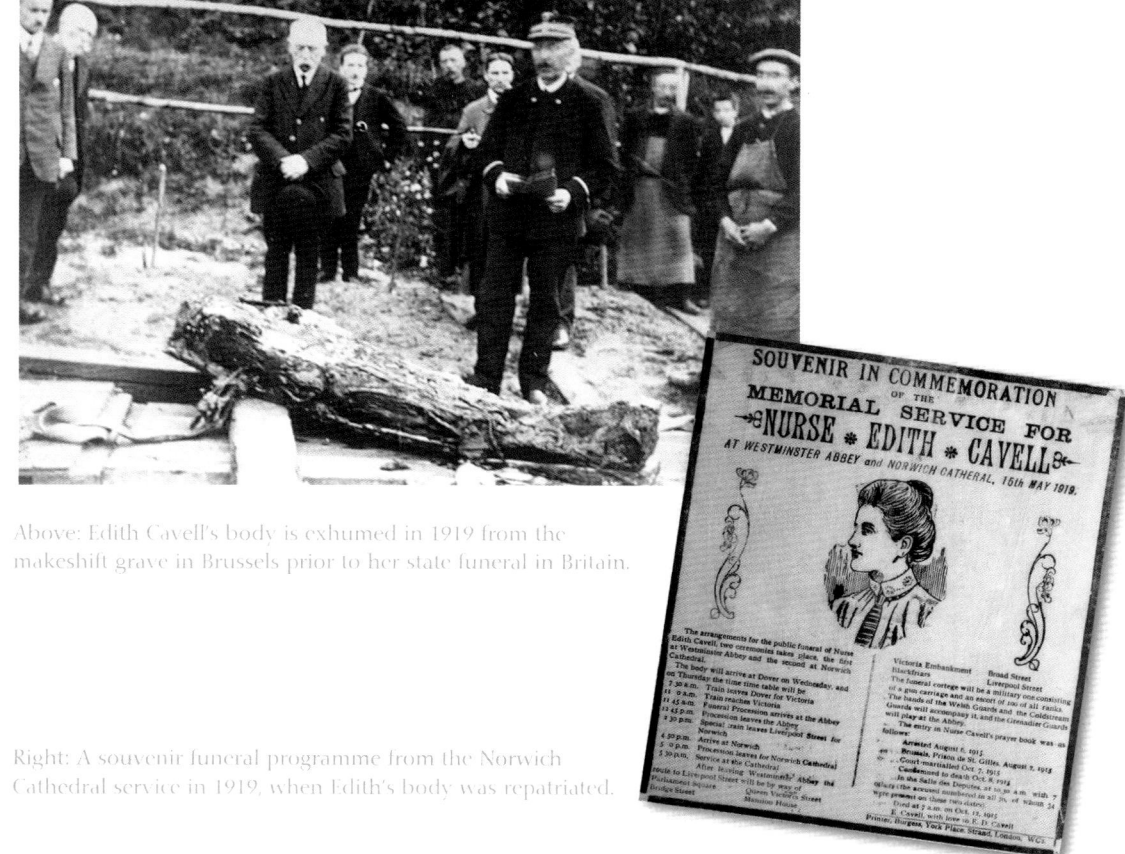

Above: Edith Cavell's body is exhumed in 1919 from the makeshift grave in Brussels prior to her state funeral in Britain.

Right: A souvenir funeral programme from the Norwich Cathedral service in 1919, when Edith's body was repatriated.

she had written to her mother, to the nurses, and to Grace Jemmett. By the cell door they shook hands. She smiled and said, 'We shall meet again'. He replied, 'Yes, we shall. God be with you'.

Edith Cavell then wrote a final letter to her deputy, Elisabeth Wilkins:

> My dear Sister
>   Mr Gahan will give you twenty francs from me to pay my little debts. Miss J. owes me (she will remember) a hundred francs. Take it to buy a clock for the new entrance hall. At the end of the daily account book you will see the Red Cross Accounts; money spent out from the School funds but not entered, which should have been covered by the two cheques I told you of and which is not entered either.
>   I am asking you to take charge of my will and a few things for me. You have been very kind my dear, and I thank you and the nurses for all you have done for me in the last ten weeks.
>   My love to you all, I am not afraid but quite happy.
>
>   Yours
>   E. Cavell
>   October 11th 1915

She had settled her accounts, written her letters, bequeathed a clock, and prepared her soul. She had been taught that 'By the grace of God' the reward for virtue was eternal life. Though the landscape of heaven was less coherently mapped and charted than the fields and lanes of rural Norfolk, in Edith Cavell's mind the terrain of each was familiar. From her earliest years the concept of God was as everyday as blackberrying and Sunday dinner. In her demanding life as a nurse she went beyond Church dogma to the meaning of quiescence. She loved and served without consideration of profit. Devotion truly was its own reward. For her cousin Edmund, whom she had told in 1895, 'I am going to do something useful. It will be something for people,' she inscribed the fly leaf of her copy of the *Imitation of Christ*:

> Arrested the 5th of August 1915
> Condemned to death 8th of October in the Salle des deputés at 10.30 am
> Died at 7 am on October the 12th 1915
> E. Cavell
> with love to E.D. Cavell

Monument to Edith Cavell in London.

Remembered

In the five decades of her life, Edith Cavell moved from being a compliant daughter in paternalistic Victorian society to qualifying as a nurse at a time when it first became a profession, rather than, as Florence Nightingale put it, 'just a job of last resort for those too old too weak or too drunk to do anything else'. In her forties she introduced professional nursing to Brussels, worked in French, in an unfamiliar culture, and became a resistance worker in order to defy wrongdoing and save lives in an unbelievably dangerous war.

After her execution she became a national hero in Britain, France and Belgium. 'Remember Edith Cavell' was used as a recruiting slogan on posters that depicted her being slain. In London the Edith Cavell War Memorial Committee was formed. The monument to her in St Martin's Place, north of Trafalgar Square, was commissioned. Four years after her execution, in May 1919, her exhumed body was brought from Brussels and she was given a State funeral, first in Westminster Abbey and then in Norwich Cathedral where she is buried.

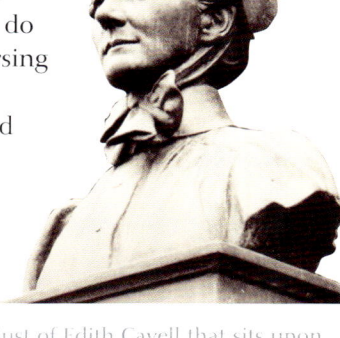

Bust of Edith Cavell that sits upon her memorial in Norwich.

In her honour other monuments were commissioned in Brussels, Paris and Norwich. Many places were named after her: streets as far away as Melbourne, Toronto and Port Louis; hospitals in Auckland, Christchurch and Brisbane; schools in British Columbia and New Brunswick; a bridge over the Shotover River near Queenstown, a mountain in Canada at Jasper National Park, a car park in Peterborough. A feature on the planet Venus was named the Cavell Corona.

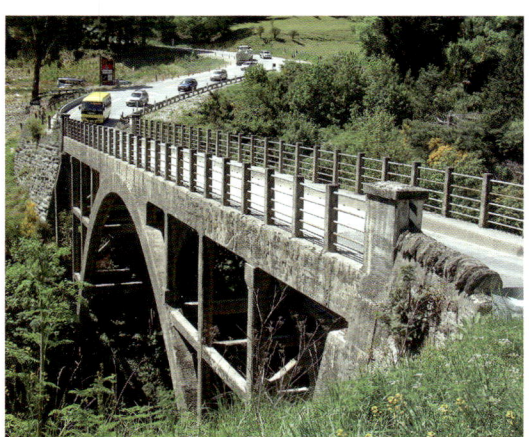

A century after her death such remembrances continue. A new headstone and setting has now been designed for her grave. Commemoration services are held yearly for her in Norwich, London and Brussels. Such actions are in honour of a nurse whose service to others and courage of heart rose above the squalor of war and injustice.

A bridge in New Zealand named after Edith Cavell.

Places to Visit

Swardeston and Norwich
Edith's birthplace and where she grew up. The church at Swardeston has a memorial stained-glass east window by E. Heaseman and holds a collection of items connected to Edith, including some of her artwork. In Norwich, in the Garden of Rest within the Cathedral Close, Edith's grave can be visited. Just outside the Cathedral Complex, opposite the Maids Head Hotel, is a memorial statue to Edith by Alfred Pegram.

London and Royal London Hospital
The hospital museum holds a collection of artefacts and images associated with Edith Cavell and has a permanent display about her. The museum also contains the chapel where Edith prayed. There is a blue plaque to Edith at the Royal London Hospital and there is a Cavell Street named after her. In St Martin's Place there is a statue in Edith's memory by George Frampton, which was unveiled by Queen Alexandra and has recently been listed as Grade I. Nurses from the Royal London Hospital in traditional uniform and representatives from Cavell Nurses' Trust and the Belgium Ambassador lay wreaths there annually. There is also a plaque to Edith in St Leonard's Hospital, Shoreditch, where Edith was assistant matron.

Peterborough Cathedral
Edith was at school in the Cathedral Close in Peterborough and in the Cathedral there is a memorial plaque to her. There are also a number of places named in her memory, including the campus of the hospital, a mental health unit and a car park.

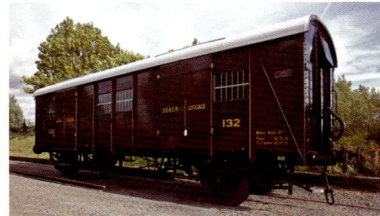

Cavell Van
This is currently at the Kent and East Sussex Railway and is the van that transported Edith's body from Belgium to London and on to Norwich to her final resting place. This van also transported the body of the 'Unknown Soldier'.

Brussels
The hospital in Uccle is named in memory of Edith Cavell and the Tir National where she was executed, on the outskirts of the city in Schaerbeek, can also be visited. At the range there is a small plaque commemorating her, as well as others who were executed during the war. There is also a monument to Edith and Depage in the city.

Manchester
Edith worked at the Sick Poor and Private Nursing Institute in Salford, Manchester, and when the matron was taken ill she took over that role. Edith is remembered on a war memorial in the grounds of Sacred Trinity Church, Salford.